OPTIMAL HEALTH THROUGH HIGH-FIBER NUTRITION

A Comprehensive Guide to Boost Digestion, Weight Management, and Longevity

Adams .U. Morris

TABLE OF CONTENTS

CHAPTER 1

High-Fiber Diet

In this opening chapter, we embark on a journey into the world of high-fiber diets. We'll break down the complex science and buzzwords, focusing on the essence of why dietary fiber matters to your health. It's the foundation upon which the rest of the book stands.

Why Should You Care About Fiber?

Imagine your body as a well-oiled machine, with numerous moving parts working together in harmony. Now, picture fiber as the maintenance crew that ensures everything runs smoothly. Fiber is a crucial part of your diet because it plays a similar role in maintaining the health and well-being of your body.

Understanding Dietary Fiber

Before we delve deeper, let's demystify the term "dietary fiber." Simply put, dietary fiber is the indigestible part of plant-based foods. It's the structural framework of fruits, vegetables, grains, nuts, and seeds that your body can't break down entirely during digestion. Instead, it travels through your digestive system largely intact, like a broom, sweeping away waste and supporting various bodily functions along the way.

There are two primary types of dietary fiber: soluble and insoluble. Think of them as a dynamic duo, each with its unique superpowers.

Soluble Fiber

Soluble fiber dissolves in water to form a gel-like substance in your digestive tract. This gel acts as a sponge, soaking up excess cholesterol and sugar, helping to regulate blood sugar levels, and lowering your risk of heart disease. You can find soluble fiber in foods like oats, beans, fruits (like apples and citrus), and vegetables.

Insoluble Fiber

On the other hand, insoluble fiber doesn't dissolve in water. It's nature's broom, adding bulk to your stool and preventing constipation. Insoluble fiber can be found in the skins of fruits and vegetables, whole grains, and nuts.

The Historical Perspective

The concept of a high-fiber diet isn't new. Our ancestors, who had diets rich in whole, unprocessed foods, naturally consumed ample amounts of fiber. However, with the advent of modern food processing, our diets have shifted significantly. We now often consume more processed foods that are stripped of their natural fiber content. This shift has come with a host of health problems, including increased rates of heart disease, diabetes, and digestive issues.

To appreciate the importance of high-fiber diets today, it's essential to understand how we got here. In recent decades, researchers and healthcare professionals have begun to reconnect with the wisdom of our ancestors, recognizing the pivotal role that dietary fiber plays in our health. As a result, high-fiber diets have gained renewed attention and popularity.

The Benefits of a High-Fiber Diet

So, why is all this fuss about fiber? The benefits are abundant and far-reaching:

1. Digestive Health: Fiber acts as a natural laxative, promoting regular bowel movements and preventing constipation. It also supports the growth of beneficial gut bacteria, contributing to a healthy gut microbiome.

2. Weight Management: If you're looking to shed a few pounds or maintain a healthy weight, fiber can be your ally. High-fiber foods are often filling and low in calories, helping you control your appetite and reduce overall calorie intake.

3. Heart Health: Soluble fiber is particularly beneficial for your heart. It can help lower LDL (bad) cholesterol levels and reduce your risk of heart disease.

4. Blood Sugar Control: For those concerned about diabetes or blood sugar spikes, fiber can help regulate blood glucose levels by slowing the absorption of sugar from the digestive tract.

5. Cancer Prevention: Some studies suggest that a high-fiber diet may reduce the risk of certain types of cancer, particularly colorectal cancer.

6. Longevity: A diet rich in fiber has been associated with a longer lifespan and a reduced risk of chronic diseases, contributing to overall vitality and well-being.

7. Gut-Brain Connection: Emerging research is uncovering the intricate relationship between gut health and mental well-being. A healthy gut, fostered by dietary fiber, may positively influence mood and cognitive function.

8. Skin Health: Believe it or not, what you eat can impact your skin's health. A fiber-rich diet can help flush out toxins and promote a clear complexion.

Closing Thoughts

In this opening chapter, we've set the stage for your journey into the world of high-fiber diets. Dietary fiber isn't just another dietary fad; it's the missing piece in many modern diets that can help restore and maintain our health.

Throughout this book, we'll explore the different types of dietary fiber, understand how they work in your body, and learn how to incorporate them into your daily meals. We'll address the challenges and offer practical solutions to make a high-fiber diet not just a short-term fix but a sustainable and enjoyable way of eating.

So, whether you're aiming to improve your digestive health, manage your weight, or simply lead a healthier life, dietary fiber is your faithful companion on this journey. Buckle up; it's going to be an enlightening ride into the world of high-fiber nutrition.

CHAPTER 2

Why Fiber Matters

In this chapter, we'll delve deep into the why of fiber. Why should you care about it? What makes it so essential to your health? Let's explore these questions and more.

The Building Blocks of Health

Imagine your body as a complex structure, much like a house. For that structure to stand strong and function optimally, it requires a solid foundation. In the context of your body, that foundation is built

from the nutrients and
components it needs to thrive, and
one of those essential building
blocks is dietary fiber.

The Role of Fiber

Dietary fiber is often described as
the unsung hero of nutrition. It
doesn't get the same glamour as
protein, carbohydrates, or healthy
fats, but it plays a pivotal role in
maintaining your health. To
understand why it matters, we
need to explore its functions.

1. Digestive Health

Fiber is like the custodian of your
digestive system. Its primary job is

to keep things moving. How? Well, think of it as a broom. As it travels through your digestive tract, it sweeps away waste, toxins, and anything that shouldn't be there. This helps prevent constipation and supports regular, healthy bowel movements.

But fiber does more than just sweep. It also promotes the growth of beneficial bacteria in your gut. These friendly microbes are essential for a well-balanced and robust digestive system. They help break down food, absorb nutrients, and even support your immune system.

2. Weight Management

If you've ever tried to manage your weight, you know how important it is to feel full and satisfied after a meal. This is where fiber shines. High-fiber foods tend to be filling, and they stay in your stomach longer than low-fiber foods. This means you're less likely to overeat or snack between meals.

Moreover, because fiber-rich foods are often lower in calories, they can help you create a calorie deficit, which is key to weight loss. You can enjoy larger portions of these foods without consuming excessive calories, making them an excellent tool for those aiming to shed extra pounds.

3. Heart Health

Your heart is one of the most vital organs in your body, and it deserves all the care and attention you can give it. This is where soluble fiber steps in. Soluble fiber, found in foods like oats, beans, and fruits, has a unique ability to lower LDL (low-density lipoprotein) cholesterol levels, often referred to as "bad" cholesterol.

When you consume soluble fiber, it forms a gel-like substance in your digestive tract. This gel binds to cholesterol molecules, preventing them from being absorbed into your bloodstream. Over time, this can help reduce your risk of heart disease, one of the leading causes of death worldwide.

4. Blood Sugar Regulation

Whether you have diabetes or simply want to maintain stable energy levels throughout the day, blood sugar control is crucial. This is where fiber, particularly soluble fiber, again comes to the rescue. When you eat foods rich in soluble fiber, they slow down the absorption of sugar from your digestive tract into your bloodstream.

This gradual release of sugar helps prevent sharp spikes and crashes in your blood sugar levels. It provides a steady supply of energy, which can help with concentration, mood stability, and overall well-being.

5. Longevity and Disease Prevention

Picture fiber as a shield, protecting your body from various health threats. A high-fiber diet has been linked to a reduced risk of chronic diseases such as diabetes, heart disease, and certain types of cancer, particularly colorectal cancer.

Moreover, studies have shown that individuals who consume more fiber tend to live longer and experience a higher quality of life in their later years. This is because fiber contributes to overall vitality and well-being by supporting various bodily functions.

6. Gut-Brain Connection

Scientists are beginning to uncover the profound connection between the gut and the brain, often referred to as the "gut-brain axis." A healthy gut, nourished by a high-fiber diet, may positively influence mood, cognitive function, and even mental health conditions like depression and anxiety.

This connection is fascinating and suggests that what you eat not only affects your physical health but also your mental and emotional well-being.

7. Skin Health

Yes, the benefits of fiber extend to your skin too. Clear, radiant skin isn't just about creams and lotions;

it starts from within. A high-fiber diet can help eliminate toxins from your body more efficiently, which can lead to a clearer complexion.

Moreover, by supporting healthy digestion and nutrient absorption, fiber ensures that your skin receives the vitamins and minerals it needs to glow.

8. The Big Picture of Health

When you piece together these individual benefits, you see the bigger picture. Fiber isn't just a single nutrient; it's a multifaceted powerhouse that contributes to your overall health and well-being.

It's the unsung hero that quietly goes about its business, keeping your body in balance.

The Bottom Line

In this chapter, we've explored why fiber matters, and it's abundantly clear that its impact on your health is profound. From promoting digestive health to aiding in weight management, from supporting heart health to regulating blood sugar, fiber plays an indispensable role.

As we continue through this book, we'll dive deeper into the practical aspects of incorporating fiber into your daily diet. You'll discover which foods are rich in fiber, how to plan fiber-packed meals, and strategies to overcome common challenges.

So, if you've ever wondered why people make such a fuss about fiber, you now have your answer. It's not just another dietary buzzword; it's the foundation upon which your health and vitality stand. It's time to embrace the power of fiber and make it an essential part of your nutritional journey.

CHAPTER 3

Types of Dietary Fiber

In this chapter, we're going to dive deep into the world of dietary fiber and explore its different types. You'll discover that dietary fiber is not a one-size-fits-all nutrient; it comes in various forms, each with its unique benefits. Let's unravel the intricacies of soluble and insoluble fiber and how they contribute to your health.

The Dynamic Duo: Soluble and Insoluble Fiber

Dietary fiber can be broadly classified into two main categories: soluble and insoluble fiber. Think of them as the dynamic duo, working together to support your health in different ways.

Soluble Fiber: The Gel Makers

Soluble fiber, as the name suggests, dissolves in water. It has a remarkable ability to transform into a gel-like substance when it comes into contact with liquids. This unique quality gives soluble fiber its distinct characteristics and health benefits.

1. Cholesterol Management

One of the standout features of soluble fiber is its role in cholesterol management. When you consume foods rich in soluble fiber, like oats, beans, and certain fruits, the soluble fiber forms a gel in your digestive tract. This gel acts like a sponge, trapping cholesterol molecules and preventing them from being absorbed into your bloodstream. Over time, this can lead to a reduction in LDL (low-density lipoprotein) cholesterol, often referred to as "bad" cholesterol. Lower LDL cholesterol levels are associated with a reduced risk of heart disease.

2. Blood Sugar Regulation

Soluble fiber also plays a crucial role in blood sugar regulation. When you eat foods rich in soluble fiber, they slow down the digestion and absorption of carbohydrates. This results in a gradual and steady release of sugar into your bloodstream, helping to prevent rapid spikes and crashes in blood sugar levels. For individuals with diabetes or those aiming to maintain stable energy levels, soluble fiber can be a valuable ally.

3. Weight Management

Soluble fiber has a satiating effect, which means it helps you feel full and satisfied after a meal. This feeling of fullness can curb overeating and snacking between meals, making it an excellent tool for weight management.

Moreover, foods high in soluble fiber tend to be low in calories. So, you can enjoy larger portions of these foods without consuming excessive calories. This combination of fullness and lower calorie intake can contribute to weight loss or weight maintenance.

Insoluble Fiber: Nature's Broom

In contrast to soluble fiber, insoluble fiber does not dissolve in water. Instead, it retains its structure as it moves through your digestive tract, acting like nature's broom.

1. Digestive Health

Insoluble fiber is your digestive system's best friend. It adds bulk to your stool, making it softer and more comfortable to pass. This can help prevent constipation and keep your bowel movements regular and healthy.

Moreover, the "roughage" provided by insoluble fiber stimulates the muscles in your intestinal walls, promoting the efficient movement of food and waste through your digestive system.

2. Weight Management

Like soluble fiber, insoluble fiber can also contribute to weight management. Foods high in insoluble fiber are often lower in calorie density, meaning they provide fewer calories for the same volume of food. This can help you feel full without overloading on calories.

3. Colon Health

Insoluble fiber has been linked to a reduced risk of certain digestive conditions, particularly colorectal cancer. This protective effect is thought to be due to the bulk and increased regularity that insoluble fiber provides to your bowel movements. Regular bowel movements can help eliminate potential carcinogens more efficiently.

Where to Find Soluble and Insoluble Fiber

Now that you understand the unique benefits of each type of

dietary fiber, let's explore where you can find them in your diet.

Sources of Soluble Fiber:

1. **Oats:** Oatmeal is a classic source of soluble fiber. It's a great way to start your day with a heart-healthy breakfast.

2. **Legumes:** Beans, lentils, and chickpeas are rich in soluble fiber and make excellent additions to soups, stews, and salads.

3. **Fruits:** Certain fruits, like apples, pears, and citrus fruits, are high in soluble

fiber. Leave the skin on for an extra fiber boost.

4. **Vegetables:** Some vegetables, such as carrots and sweet potatoes, contain soluble fiber. Plus, they're loaded with vitamins and minerals.

5. **Nuts and Seeds:** Almonds, flaxseeds, and chia seeds are nutritious sources of soluble fiber. They can be sprinkled on yogurt or added to smoothies.

Sources of Insoluble Fiber:

1. **Whole Grains:** Whole wheat, brown rice, quinoa,

and whole-grain bread and pasta are excellent sources of insoluble fiber. Opt for whole grains over refined grains for added fiber.

2. **Vegetables:** Many vegetables, including broccoli, cauliflower, and dark leafy greens, are rich in insoluble fiber. They add texture and flavor to your meals.

3. **Fruit Skins:** Don't peel your fruits; instead, consume them with the skin intact. This includes fruits like apples, pears, and grapes.

4. **Nuts and Seeds:** These are not only sources of soluble fiber but also insoluble fiber. They can be incorporated into a variety of dishes for added crunch and nutrition.

Balancing Your Fiber Intake

A well-rounded, healthy diet includes both soluble and insoluble fiber. Together, they create a harmonious balance that supports your digestive health, weight management, and overall well-being.

However, it's essential to increase your fiber intake gradually.

Sudden and significant changes in your fiber intake can lead to digestive discomfort, such as gas and bloating. Instead, make small, incremental adjustments to your diet to allow your digestive system time to adapt.

In the next chapters, we'll delve into practical strategies for incorporating these fiber-rich foods into your meals and snacks. We'll also address common challenges and provide solutions to help you maintain a high-fiber diet comfortably and sustainably.

In summary, dietary fiber isn't a one-size-fits-all nutrient. Soluble and insoluble fiber each have their unique roles in supporting your health. By understanding these distinctions and incorporating a variety of fiber-rich foods into your diet, you can harness the full spectrum of fiber's benefits for your well-being.

CHAPTER 4

Fiber and Digestive Health

Welcome to the fascinating world of digestive health and fiber! In this chapter, we're going to take a deep dive into how fiber plays a crucial role in maintaining a healthy digestive system. Think of fiber as your digestive system's best friend, always there to keep things running smoothly.

The Digestive System: Your Body's Processing Plant

Before we explore the relationship between fiber and digestive health, let's take a moment to understand the digestive system itself. Think of it as a complex processing plant responsible for breaking down the foods you eat into nutrients your body can use.

The journey starts in your mouth, where enzymes in your saliva begin to break down carbohydrates. From there, your food travels down your esophagus and into your stomach, where it's mixed with stomach acid to further break down proteins.

Next stop: the small intestine. This is where the magic happens. Nutrients are absorbed through the lining of the small intestine and transported to various parts of your body through your bloodstream.

But what about the parts of your food that can't be broken down and absorbed, like fiber? This is where fiber's role becomes critical.

Fiber: Nature's Broom

Dietary fiber is like the janitor of your digestive system. It's the part of plant-based foods that your body can't fully digest or absorb.

Instead, fiber continues its journey through your digestive tract largely intact, performing some vital tasks along the way.

1. Promoting Regularity

One of the primary roles of fiber is to add bulk to your stool, making it softer and easier to pass. This can help prevent constipation, a common digestive issue characterized by infrequent and difficult bowel movements.

Picture fiber as a gentle, natural laxative. As it moves through your intestines, it absorbs water and adds moisture to your stool, preventing it from becoming too hard and dry. This makes for more comfortable and regular bowel movements.

2. Preventing Diverticulosis

Diverticulosis is a condition in which small pouches (diverticula) form in the wall of your colon. These pouches can become inflamed or infected, leading to diverticulitis, a more severe condition.

Fiber plays a protective role here. A high-fiber diet can help prevent diverticulosis by keeping your stool soft and bulky, which reduces pressure on the colon walls. This, in turn, lowers the risk of diverticula formation.

3. Supporting a Healthy Gut Microbiome

Inside your intestines resides a bustling community of microorganisms known as your gut microbiome. These tiny inhabitants play a significant role in your overall health, from aiding digestion to influencing your immune system and even your mood.

Fiber is like their preferred food source. It reaches your colon largely undigested, where it becomes a feast for your gut bacteria. These bacteria ferment fiber, breaking it down into substances like short-chain fatty acids, which have numerous health benefits.

4. Preventing Colon Cancer

There's mounting evidence that a high-fiber diet may reduce the risk of colon cancer, one of the most common types of cancer worldwide. The exact mechanisms aren't fully understood, but it's thought to be related to the protective effects of fiber on the colon.

By promoting regular bowel movements, maintaining a healthy gut environment, and reducing inflammation, fiber may help lower the risk of colon cancer.

5. Managing Irritable Bowel Syndrome (IBS)

Irritable Bowel Syndrome, or IBS, is a chronic digestive disorder characterized by symptoms like abdominal pain, bloating, and changes in bowel habits. While the causes of IBS are complex and multifaceted, some individuals find relief through dietary adjustments, including increasing their fiber intake.

However, it's important to note that IBS is highly individual, and what works for one person may not work for another. Some individuals with IBS may need to be cautious with certain types of fiber, while others may benefit from it.

Balancing Fiber Intake

While fiber offers numerous digestive benefits, it's essential to strike a balance. Too much fiber, especially if you increase your intake suddenly, can lead to digestive discomfort, including gas and bloating.

Here are some tips for achieving a balanced fiber intake:

1. Gradual Increase: If you're not used to a high-fiber diet, introduce fiber-rich foods gradually. This gives your digestive system time to adjust.

2. Hydration: Fiber absorbs water, so be sure to drink plenty of fluids throughout the day to help fiber move smoothly through your digestive tract.

3. Variety: Consume a variety of fiber-rich foods to get the full spectrum of benefits from different types of fiber.

4. Listen to Your Body: Pay attention to how your body reacts to different foods. Everyone's digestive system is unique, and what works for one person may not work for another.

Practical Tips for a High-Fiber Diet

In the upcoming chapters, we'll delve into practical strategies for incorporating fiber-rich foods into your daily meals and snacks. You'll learn how to plan balanced, fiber-packed meals and find creative ways to enjoy the full range of fiber's benefits.

In summary, fiber is a key player in maintaining a healthy digestive system. From preventing constipation to supporting your gut microbiome and reducing the risk of colon cancer, fiber's contributions are invaluable. By embracing fiber as nature's broom and gradually increasing your intake, you can reap the rewards of a well-functioning digestive system.

CHAPTER 5

Fiber and Weight Management

In this chapter, we embark on a journey to understand how fiber plays a pivotal role in weight management. Fiber is like a silent partner in your quest for a healthier weight, and its impact goes far beyond just filling your stomach. Let's explore why fiber matters in the context of weight management and how it can be your ally on this journey.

The Complex Landscape of Weight Management

Before we dive into the specifics of fiber's role in weight management, it's essential to grasp the complexity of weight control. Weight management isn't solely about shedding pounds; it's about achieving and maintaining a healthy balance that works for your body.

Weight management involves a multitude of factors, including genetics, metabolism, physical activity, hormones, and, of course, diet. And within the realm of diet, fiber emerges as a powerful tool that can influence various aspects of your weight management journey.

Fiber and Satiety: Feeling Full and Satisfied

One of the primary ways fiber contributes to weight management is by promoting satiety. Satiety is the feeling of fullness and satisfaction you experience after eating a meal. It's the signal your body sends to your brain to indicate that you've had enough to eat.

Fiber-rich foods have a remarkable ability to enhance

satiety. When you consume foods high in fiber, they take longer to chew and digest, giving your body more time to register that you're full. This slower digestion also leads to a gradual and sustained release of nutrients into your bloodstream, helping you maintain stable energy levels and avoid the energy crashes associated with high-sugar, low-fiber foods.

The Role of Fiber's Texture

The texture of fiber-rich foods also contributes to their satiating effect. Foods like whole grains, vegetables, and fruits often require more chewing, which can slow down your eating pace. This slower pace gives your body more time to send satiety signals, helping you avoid overeating.

Calorie Density: More Food, Fewer Calories

Another fascinating aspect of fiber-rich foods is their calorie density. Calorie density refers to the number of calories in a given volume of food. Foods that are high in fiber tend to have lower calorie density, meaning they provide fewer calories for the same volume of food.

This characteristic is particularly valuable for those looking to control their calorie intake. You can enjoy larger portions of fiber-rich foods without consuming excessive calories. In other words, fiber allows you to eat more food while still managing your calorie intake effectively.

Fiber and Appetite Control

Beyond its physical attributes, fiber also has an impact on your appetite control mechanisms. Some studies suggest that fiber can influence the release of hormones that regulate hunger and fullness. For instance, it may stimulate the production of hormones like cholecystokinin (CCK) and glucagon-like peptide-1 (GLP-1), which help reduce appetite.

Moreover, fiber-rich foods often require more effort to eat, which can lead to greater mindfulness during meals. This increased awareness of what you're eating can help you tune in to your body's hunger and fullness cues, reducing the likelihood of overeating.

Practical Tips for Using Fiber in Weight Management

Now that you understand how fiber supports weight management, let's explore some practical tips for incorporating fiber into your daily diet to achieve your weight-related goals:

1. Start Your Day Right: Begin your mornings with a fiber-rich breakfast. Whole-grain cereal, oatmeal, or a smoothie with added fruits and vegetables are excellent choices.

2. Include Fiber in Every Meal: Aim to include fiber-rich foods in every meal. Add veggies to your sandwiches and wraps, opt for whole grains like brown rice or quinoa, and snack on fruits and nuts.

3. Embrace Fiber-Rich Snacks: When snacking, choose options that provide both fiber and protein, as this combination can enhance satiety. Examples include apple slices with almond butter or Greek yogurt with berries.

4. Gradual Changes: If you're new to a high-fiber diet, introduce fiber-rich foods gradually. Sudden increases in fiber intake can lead to digestive discomfort, such as gas and bloating.

5. Hydration: Fiber absorbs water, so be sure to drink plenty of fluids throughout the day. Staying hydrated supports the proper function of fiber in your digestive system.

6. Read Labels: When shopping for packaged foods, read the labels. Look for products that list whole grains, fruits, and vegetables as their primary ingredients. Pay attention to the fiber content per serving.

7. Mindful Eating: Practice mindful eating by savoring your meals and paying attention to your body's hunger and fullness cues.

Avoid distractions like screens during mealtimes.

The Long-Term Perspective

It's essential to approach weight management with a long-term perspective. Fiber is not a quick-fix solution for weight loss; rather, it's a sustainable and healthful approach to achieving and maintaining a healthy weight over time.

By incorporating fiber-rich foods into your diet, you can create a foundation for balanced eating habits that support your overall well-being. Remember that weight management is not solely about the number on the scale but about nurturing a healthy relationship with food and your body.

In the chapters ahead, we'll explore more practical strategies for making fiber a consistent and enjoyable part of your diet. We'll also address common challenges and provide solutions to help you succeed in your weight management journey.

In summary, fiber is a valuable ally in your quest for weight management. Its satiating effects, ability to reduce calorie density, and impact on appetite control make it a powerful tool. By gradually increasing your fiber intake and making fiber-rich foods a regular part of your meals and snacks, you can harness the benefits of fiber for sustainable weight management.

Chapter 6: Meal Planning for a High-Fiber Diet

In this chapter, we step into the practical realm of meal planning for a high-fiber diet. You've learned about the benefits of fiber, its role in digestive health and weight management, and now it's time to put that knowledge into action. Let's explore how to design balanced, satisfying, and fiber-rich meals that nourish your body.

The Art of Meal Planning

Meal planning is like having a blueprint for your nutritional success. It involves thoughtful preparation and organization of your meals to ensure that you meet your dietary goals, whether it's increasing your fiber intake, managing your weight, or promoting overall well-being.

Here's a step-by-step guide to meal planning for a high-fiber diet:

1. Assess Your Current Diet:

Start by taking stock of your current eating habits. What does a typical day of meals look like for you? This self-assessment can help you identify areas where you can incorporate more fiber-rich foods.

2. Set Realistic Goals:

Set specific, achievable goals for your high-fiber diet. For example, you might aim to consume a certain number of grams of fiber per day or incorporate a particular fiber-rich food into each meal.

3. Choose a Variety of Fiber Sources:

Dietary diversity is key to ensuring you get a wide range of nutrients and benefits. Select a variety of fiber sources from different food groups. This includes fruits, vegetables, whole grains, legumes, nuts, and seeds.

4. Plan Your Meals:

Create a weekly meal plan that includes breakfast, lunch, dinner, and snacks. Incorporate fiber-rich foods into each meal to spread your fiber intake throughout the day. For example:

- **Breakfast:** Start your day with a bowl of oatmeal topped with fresh berries and a sprinkle of chia seeds. Alternatively, enjoy a veggie-packed omelet with whole-grain toast.
- **Lunch:** Opt for a salad filled with leafy greens, colorful vegetables, chickpeas, and a

drizzle of olive oil and balsamic vinegar. Pair it with a serving of quinoa or brown rice.

- **Dinner:** Prepare a stir-fry with tofu or lean protein and a medley of broccoli, bell peppers, and snap peas. Serve it over brown rice or whole-grain noodles.

- **Snacks:** Reach for fiber-rich snacks like carrot sticks with hummus, a piece of fruit, or a small handful of mixed nuts.

5. Be Mindful of Portion Sizes:

While fiber-rich foods are nutritious, portion control is still essential, especially if you're managing your weight. Pay attention to recommended serving sizes to avoid overeating.

6. Meal Prep:

Consider batch cooking and meal prepping to save time during the week. Cook large quantities of grains, beans, and vegetables that can be used in various meals.

7. Experiment with Recipes:

Don't be afraid to get creative with your meals. Try new recipes that feature fiber-rich ingredients.

Explore the world of cuisines, as many international dishes incorporate high-fiber foods.

8. Stay Hydrated:

Remember to drink plenty of water throughout the day. Fiber absorbs water, and staying hydrated helps fiber move smoothly through your digestive system.

9. Listen to Your Body:

Pay attention to your body's hunger and fullness cues. Eat when you're hungry, and stop when you're satisfied. Mindful eating can help you maintain a healthy relationship with food.

10. Monitor Your Progress:

Keep a food diary to track your fiber intake and how your body responds. This can help you fine-tune your meal planning and make adjustments as needed.

The Balanced Plate: A High-Fiber Approach

One effective way to ensure that your meals are high in fiber is to create a balanced plate. Imagine dividing your plate into sections, each dedicated to specific food groups:

1. **Vegetables:** Fill half your plate with non-starchy vegetables like leafy greens, broccoli, carrots, peppers, and cauliflower. These veggies are low in calories but high in fiber, vitamins, and minerals.

2. **Whole Grains:** Allocate a quarter of your plate to whole grains like brown rice, quinoa, whole wheat pasta, or whole-grain bread. These grains provide complex carbohydrates and additional fiber.

3. **Lean Protein:** The remaining quarter of your plate can be reserved for lean protein sources, such as beans, lentils, tofu,

skinless poultry, or fish. Protein helps keep you feeling full and satisfied.

4. Healthy Fats: Don't forget to include healthy fats in your meal, such as avocados, nuts, seeds, and olive oil. These fats provide essential nutrients and add flavor to your dishes.

5. Fruit: While not on your plate, fruit can be an excellent addition to your meal or enjoyed as a dessert. Berries, apples, pears, and citrus fruits are particularly high in fiber.

Fiber-Rich Meal Ideas

Let's put these principles into practice with some fiber-rich meal ideas:

1. Fiber-Packed Breakfast:

- Greek yogurt parfait with layers of berries, whole-grain granola, and a drizzle of honey.

2. Hearty Lunch:

- Spinach and kale salad with chickpeas, roasted sweet potatoes, quinoa, and a tahini dressing.

3. Nutrient-Rich Dinner:

- Baked salmon with a side of steamed broccoli and a quinoa pilaf with mixed vegetables.

4. Satisfying Snack:

- Sliced cucumbers and cherry tomatoes with a side of hummus.

5. Sweet Treat:

- Baked apple with cinnamon and a sprinkle of chopped walnuts.

In these examples, you can see how different meals can be designed with a variety of high-fiber foods. The key is to keep your meals balanced, colorful, and satisfying.

A Sustainable Approach

Remember that meal planning for a high-fiber diet is not about quick fixes or rigid rules. It's about cultivating a sustainable and healthful way of eating that supports your well-being over the long term. By gradually incorporating fiber-rich foods into your meals and paying attention to portion sizes and hunger cues, you can embrace a high-fiber diet as a practical and enjoyable lifestyle choice.

In the upcoming chapters, we'll continue to explore practical strategies and address common challenges to help you succeed on your high-fiber journey. Whether you're aiming for better digestive health, weight management, or overall vitality, meal planning plays a vital role in achieving your goals.

CHAPTER 7

Overcoming Common Challenges in a High-Fiber Diet

Congratulations on your journey to embrace a high-fiber diet! As you've learned, the benefits of fiber are abundant, from supporting digestive health to aiding in weight management. However, like any lifestyle change, adopting a high-fiber diet can come with its challenges. In this chapter, we'll explore these common hurdles and provide practical solutions to help you overcome them.

Challenge 1: Digestive Discomfort

One of the most frequently reported challenges when increasing fiber intake is digestive discomfort. Gas, bloating, and changes in bowel habits can occur, especially if you make sudden and significant changes to your diet.

Solution: Gradual Increase

The key to mitigating digestive discomfort is a gradual increase in fiber. Instead of drastically increasing your fiber intake overnight, make small, incremental changes to your diet. Your digestive system needs time to adapt to the additional fiber.

Start by adding a single high-fiber food item to one meal each day. Over the course of a few weeks, gradually introduce more fiber-rich foods. This gentle approach can help your digestive system adjust without causing discomfort.

Challenge 2: Lack of Variety

Another challenge can be falling into a routine of eating the same high-fiber foods repeatedly. This lack of variety can lead to boredom and make it difficult to sustain a high-fiber diet in the long run.

Solution: Explore New Foods and Recipes

Embrace variety in your high-fiber diet by exploring new foods and recipes. There's an abundance of fiber-rich foods to choose from, so take advantage of this diversity.

- **Try Different Grains:** Experiment with grains like quinoa, farro, bulgur, and barley in place of your usual rice or pasta.

- **Explore Legumes:** Discover the world of

legumes, including lentils, chickpeas, black beans, and pinto beans. They can be used in soups, stews, salads, and even as burger alternatives.

- **Fruits and Veggies:** Seasonal fruits and vegetables provide an ever-changing array of flavors and nutrients. Visit local farmers' markets for inspiration.

- **Spices and Herbs:** Elevate your dishes with a variety of herbs and spices to keep your meals exciting and flavorful.

Challenge 3: Social and Dining Out Pressures

Social situations and dining out can present challenges when you're committed to a high-fiber diet. Restaurant menus and social gatherings may not always offer fiber-rich options.

Solution: Plan Ahead and Communicate

Planning ahead is crucial in these situations. Before dining out, check the restaurant's menu online to identify fiber-rich choices. Many restaurants now offer dietary information on their websites.

If you're attending a social event, communicate your dietary preferences or restrictions to the host. You can offer to bring a dish that aligns with your high-fiber goals, ensuring you have a suitable option.

When ordering at a restaurant, don't hesitate to customize your meal to include more fiber-rich ingredients. For example, ask for extra veggies in your stir-fry or swap out white rice for brown rice.

Challenge 4: Time Constraints

In today's fast-paced world, finding the time to prepare fiber-rich meals can be a challenge. Convenience foods often lack the fiber content your diet requires.

Solution: Meal Prep and Quick Fixes

Meal prepping can be a lifesaver when you have a busy schedule. Dedicate some time each week to prepare and store fiber-rich components like cooked grains, roasted vegetables, and pre-washed greens. This way, you can assemble quick, balanced meals on the go.

Additionally, keep a stash of fiber-rich snacks on hand for those moments when you need a quick fix. Portable options like nuts, seeds, whole fruit, or whole-grain crackers can tide you over until your next meal.

Challenge 5: Texture and Taste Preferences

Some individuals may find the texture or taste of certain high-fiber foods unappealing. For example, the texture of cooked beans or the taste of whole-grain bread may not align with everyone's palate.

Solution: Experiment and Adapt

Fiber-rich foods come in a wide range of textures and flavors. If you're not a fan of a particular fiber source, don't give up on it altogether. Experiment with different cooking methods, seasonings, and recipes to find a preparation that suits your taste.

For example, if you're not fond of plain cooked beans, try making a flavorful bean salad or blending them into soups for a smoother texture. Similarly, whole grains can be incorporated into dishes where their taste complements other ingredients.

Challenge 6: Travel and On-the-Go Eating

Traveling or being constantly on the move can disrupt your high-fiber routine. Fast food and convenience store snacks may seem like the only options.

Solution: Portable Fiber Sources

Pack travel-friendly fiber-rich snacks for your journeys. Nuts, seeds, dried fruit, and whole-grain crackers can be easily stashed in your bag.

Additionally, seek out healthier options at airports, gas stations, or rest stops. Many places now offer prepackaged salads, yogurt with granola, or fruit cups that can help you maintain your fiber intake while on the go.

Challenge 7: Fiber Myths and Misconceptions

Sometimes, myths and misconceptions about fiber can lead to confusion and frustration. People may hear conflicting advice or be unsure about how much fiber they actually need.

Solution: Educate Yourself

Arm yourself with accurate information about fiber. The recommended daily intake varies depending on factors like age, gender, and activity level, but a general guideline is around 25 grams for adult women and 38 grams for adult men.

Remember that fiber is a vital part of a healthy diet, and its benefits are well-documented. It's not just about preventing constipation; it plays a significant role in overall health, including heart health, weight management, and digestive well-being.

Challenge 8: Staying Consistent

Consistency is key to reaping the long-term benefits of a high-fiber diet. It's easy to fall off track when life gets busy or when cravings for less nutritious foods strike.

Solution: Prioritize and Create Habits

Make fiber-rich foods a priority in your diet by building them into your daily routine. Create habits that support your high-fiber goals, such as starting your day with a fiber-rich breakfast, keeping a bowl of fruit on your kitchen counter, or always having a container of chopped veggies in your fridge for snacking.

Remember that it's okay to indulge occasionally in less-fiber-rich foods. The key is balance and consistency over the long term.

Conclusion: Embrace the Journey

Overcoming challenges in a high-fiber diet is part of the journey toward a healthier and more balanced life. As you encounter obstacles, view them as opportunities to learn and grow in your nutritional choices.

By gradually increasing your fiber intake, embracing variety in your meals, and finding practical solutions to common challenges, you're well on your way to reaping the rewards of a high-fiber diet. Continue to explore and enjoy the many delicious and nutritious fiber-rich foods available to you, and remember that every step forward is a step toward better health and well-being.

CHAPTER 8

Maintaining a High-Fiber Diet for Life

Congratulations! You've embarked on a journey to embrace a high-fiber diet, and you've overcome common challenges along the way. Now, in this final chapter, we'll explore the key principles for maintaining a high-fiber diet for life. It's not just about a short-term change; it's about making fiber an integral part of your long-term, sustainable eating habits.

The Long-Term Perspective

Maintaining a high-fiber diet for life involves adopting a sustainable approach that becomes second nature. It's not about quick fixes or temporary solutions; it's about creating lasting, healthful habits that support your well-being.

Let's delve into the key principles for sustaining your high-fiber diet over the long term:

1. Make It a Lifestyle, Not a Diet

The first step in maintaining a high-fiber diet is to shift your mindset. Rather than viewing it as a restrictive diet, think of it as a lifestyle choice that supports your health. This perspective change can help you approach dietary decisions with a more positive and sustainable mindset.

2. Continue to Embrace Variety

Variety is the spice of life, and it's a fundamental aspect of a high-fiber diet. Continue to explore new foods, recipes, and cuisines. The world of fiber-rich foods is vast, and there's always something new to discover.

Regularly rotate your menu to ensure you get a wide range of nutrients and flavors. Experiment with seasonal produce, grains, and legumes to keep your meals exciting and enjoyable.

3. Plan and Prepare

Meal planning and preparation play a significant role in maintaining a high-fiber diet. Continue to set aside time each week to plan your meals, create shopping lists, and prepare components of your dishes in advance.

When you have fiber-rich ingredients readily available, you're more likely to incorporate them into your meals. Batch cooking and meal prepping can save time and make it easier to enjoy fiber-rich meals even on busy days.

4. Listen to Your Body

Your body is an excellent guide when it comes to maintaining a high-fiber diet. Pay attention to hunger and fullness cues. Eat when you're hungry, and stop when you're satisfied.

Mindful eating is a valuable tool for staying in tune with your body's needs. Avoid distractions during meals, savor the flavors, and appreciate the nourishment that fiber-rich foods provide.

5. Stay Hydrated

Hydration is a critical component of your high-fiber diet. Fiber absorbs water, so it's essential to drink enough fluids throughout the day. Water helps fiber move smoothly through your digestive system, preventing issues like constipation.

Make it a habit to keep a water bottle with you, and aim to drink water consistently throughout the day. Herbal teas and infused water can also contribute to your daily fluid intake.

6. Educate Yourself

Knowledge is a powerful tool in maintaining a high-fiber diet. Continue to educate yourself about the benefits of fiber and its role in supporting your health.

Stay informed about the latest research and dietary guidelines related to fiber. Understanding the science behind fiber's positive effects can reinforce your commitment to a high-fiber lifestyle.

7. Celebrate Successes, Learn from Challenges

Maintaining any dietary change can be challenging at times. Celebrate your successes and milestones along the way. Recognize and acknowledge your achievements, whether it's reaching a fiber intake goal, trying a new fiber-rich recipe, or consistently making high-fiber choices.

At the same time, learn from challenges and setbacks. If you encounter obstacles or slip into old habits, view them as opportunities for growth and improvement.

Reflect on what led to the challenge and brainstorm strategies to overcome it in the future.

8. Be Flexible and Adaptable

Life is dynamic, and circumstances change. Being flexible and adaptable is crucial in maintaining a high-fiber diet for life. There will be times when you may face unexpected challenges, such as travel, illness, or changes in your routine.

During such times, be open to making temporary adjustments while keeping your long-term goals in mind. You can find creative ways to incorporate fiber-rich foods even in challenging situations.

9. Share the Journey

Maintaining a high-fiber diet can be more enjoyable when you share the journey with others. Whether it's with family, friends, or an online community, connecting with like-minded individuals can provide support, inspiration, and motivation.

Share your successes, challenges, and favorite fiber-rich recipes with others. You may even inspire those around you to adopt healthier dietary habits.

10. Reflect on Your Progress

Regularly reflect on your progress in maintaining a high-fiber diet. Take time to assess how it has positively impacted your health, energy levels, and overall well-being.

Keep a journal to record your achievements and how you've overcome challenges. This reflection can reinforce your commitment to a high-fiber lifestyle and remind you of the positive changes it has brought to your life.

CONCLUSION

A Lifetime of Wellness

Maintaining a high-fiber diet for life is a commitment to your long-term health and well-being. It's about nurturing a positive relationship with food, embracing variety, and prioritizing nutrient-rich choices.

By making it a lifestyle, staying informed, and continually exploring the world of fiber-rich foods, you're not just adopting a diet; you're choosing a lifetime of wellness. You're investing in your health and setting the stage for a future filled with vitality and vitality.

As you continue on your high-fiber journey, remember that every choice you make is a step toward a healthier and more vibrant life. Celebrate your successes, learn from your experiences, and savor the nourishment that a high-fiber diet provides. May your path be filled with delicious meals, digestive well-being, and the many benefits that fiber has to offer.

In conclusion, your journey through the chapters of this book on a high-fiber diet has been an exploration of the numerous benefits and practical aspects of embracing fiber as a fundamental part of your dietary lifestyle. Here's a brief recap of the key takeaways:

Chapter 1: We began by understanding the digestive system and how fiber is like nature's broom, promoting regularity, preventing diverticulosis, supporting a healthy gut microbiome, preventing colon cancer, and potentially aiding in managing irritable bowel syndrome (IBS).

Chapter 2: We explored the relationship between fiber and weight management. Fiber's satiating effects, calorie density, and impact on appetite control make it a valuable tool in achieving and maintaining a healthy weight.

Chapter 3: We delved into the practical aspects of incorporating fiber into your diet. Meal planning with a focus on balance, portion control, and variety is essential to ensure you get the full range of fiber's benefits.

Chapter 4: We discussed the common challenges of a high-fiber diet and provided practical solutions for overcoming them.

Challenges such as digestive discomfort, lack of variety, social pressures, time constraints, texture and taste preferences, travel, myths and misconceptions, and staying consistent can all be addressed with the right strategies.

Chapter 5: We emphasized the importance of maintaining a long-term perspective on your high-fiber journey. It's not a short-term diet but a sustainable lifestyle choice that supports your overall well-being. The key principles include making it a lifestyle, embracing variety, planning and preparing, listening to your body, staying hydrated, educating yourself, celebrating successes, learning from challenges, being flexible, sharing the journey, and reflecting on your progress.

Chapter 6: We highlighted the significance of creating a balanced plate with a variety of high-fiber foods, including vegetables, whole grains, lean protein, and healthy fats. This approach ensures that your meals are satisfying, nutritious, and fiber-rich.

Chapter 7: We explored the practical strategies for meal planning on a high-fiber diet, considering your goals, dietary preferences, and lifestyle. By making fiber-rich foods a regular part of your meals and snacks, you can enjoy the benefits of fiber without feeling deprived.

Chapter 8: We concluded by emphasizing that maintaining a high-fiber diet is a commitment to a lifetime of wellness. It's about nurturing a positive relationship with food, staying informed, being adaptable, and enjoying the journey towards better health.

In the end, a high-fiber diet isn't just about improving your physical health; it's about embracing a holistic approach to well-being. It's about nourishing your body, promoting digestive health, managing your weight, and setting the stage for a vibrant and fulfilling life.

As you continue your high-fiber journey, remember that every choice you make in favor of fiber is a step towards better health and a future filled with vitality. May your path be filled with delicious meals, digestive well-being, and the many benefits that fiber has to offer.